Skinnygal

SMOOTHIES

Lose up to 20 Pounds in 14 Days

Copyright © 2018 by James Bowman

James Bowman

Table of Contents

Introduction

Conclusion

1

Why You Should Read This Book

Are you looking for the most efficient way to eat healthy and lose fat but still have some fun with it?

Turns out the solution is not some magic pills or powders. Read on to discover how drinking healthy smoothies can help you to feel full and eat less, and even stop you from gaining more weight!

But that's not all…

Here's what I discovered over the last few years, experimenting a lot with making my own nutritious smoothies, to help me stay in peak condition - physical and mental.

It may come as a bit of a surprise to you, but smoothies are an easy way to lose weight. You don't even need to use them as meal replacements if you're clever with your choice of ingredients.

When looking for the right tasty addition to a smoothie, fruits like berries are a secret weight loss weapon.

This is because of flavonoids, which has been shown in studies to be one of the keys for not gaining extra weight. It is even suspected that blueberries can actually stop fat cells from developing.
Other things that are great for burning extra calories include green vegetables like kale, broccoli and red peppers.

To get the most fat burning potential from your smoothies, be sure to include lots of protein rich foods that will fill you up (more on that later!) so you won't ruin your hard work by snacking later on.

Make sure your next smoothie is filled with delicious fat burning fruit and veg and you're well on your way to maintaining a healthy weight and even lose some pounds into the bargain!

Stay Hydrated

Drinking the recommended 6-8 glasses of water can seem daunting but with smoothies, you're already part of the way there.

We can get some of our water intake from our food and this includes smoothies, not least because lots of fruits and vegetables are quite rich in water.

Tip: you can make smoothies count even more for your water intake by starting the day, with a milk-based or water based version. This is a lot more hydrating than coffee, and the milk gives a nice calcium boost.

Keeps You Fuller For Longer

If you find yourself snacking because you never feel full, the fiber in fruit or veg based smoothies could be your new best friend!

Avocado is one example of a smoothie that will leave you sated until lunchtime and curb your urge to snack and you only need half an avocado to get its benefits.

You'll get a deliciously thick and creamy smoothie that's full of healthy fats, fiber and protein. The end result? You'll be full all morning!

Speaking of protein, this is another good move for eating less and losing weight. You'll also stay fuller if you load up on protein heavy smoothies, especially at breakfast time. This helps you to eat less calories as your day progresses.

For a big protein boost, pack your smoothies with things like spinach, Greek yogurt, hemp protein, cottage cheese and almonds.

Reduce Cravings for Junk Food

Drinking a protein rich smoothie to start the day is the perfect way to stop cravings and keep your appetite in check until your next meal. This will help ☐with your goal of being in shape!

If you're looking for the easiest way to consume a good amount of protein, Spinach is one of the best things to put in a smoothie. Mostly because it contains thylakoids which lessens your appetite.

Better Digestion

Have you tried the genre of smoothies called "Green smoothies"? The kind of smoothies blending fresh leafy green vegetables like spinach, kale, celery or collard.

These greens in particular are alkaline foods so they are your best bet to counteract the discomfort of acid reflux and heartburn.
Feel free to throw in some other alkaline foods such as carrots, strawberries and blueberries to the ultimate in health benefits.

A Ton of Antioxidants

A lot has been said about the importance of antioxidants in preventing heart disease, cancer and other diseases.

How can a smoothie help?

Add one to two teaspoons of Matcha green tea powder to your smoothies and you'll get a big helping of antioxidants.
In fact, these two teaspoons in your smoothie contain a whopping 10 times more antioxidants than green tea!

But that's not all…

Amongst other benefits, this can help with losing body fat. It also boosts your metabolism by several per-cent.
Other foods rich in antioxidants that you can add to your smoothies include grapes, blueberries, dark green vegetables and sweet potatoes.

Immunity Booster

Fruits and vegetables are a great source of nutrients and antioxidants for good health but some are proven to increase your immunity.

Adding sweet potato to your smoothies isn't just a way to make them taste nice; the beta-carotene that they contain is an immunity booster.

An added bonus - it's also good for your eyes and bones.

The purple variety has been shown to have promising effects for increasing immune response in chickens.
You can use sweet potato as a smoothie base but you'll also want to add in other ingredients to get the taste you want.

Better Rest

With the right ingredients, smoothies can help you to get a good night's sleep.

Other good sleep aids include kiwis and bananas.

Want to up your sleep potential that little bit more? Throw in some oats too. They contain magnesium and calcium, which studies have shown to be beneficial for superior sleep.

Natural Body Detox

Because smoothies contain so many nutritious ingredients, they can be a great way to detox your system and get rid of toxins. And because you won't be snacking, you won't be putting lots of toxins into your body either.

Some fruits and vegetables are particularly detoxifying such as garlic, papaya and beets. They can help to cleanse your blood and help the liver to get rid of toxins more efficiently. Be sure to include these goodies in some of your smoothies for the ultimate detox drink!

Makes You Feel Happy

You'll often hear people say that they feel much happier and energetic while drinking smoothies and this can be the same for you too.
Getting lots of portions of fruit and veges into your day makes you feel good and makes you more positive about your life - that's proven scientifically.

Increases Calcium Intake

You can use water (filtered or spring water) as a base for smoothies but why do that when you can pack even more nutrients in by using something else?

Using dairy based smoothies is an easy to boost your calcium intake, as well as getting vital vitamins and minerals. Calcium is an important mineral for good health and plays some key roles in the body.

Besides milk, you can use kefir from milk to provide a thick, creamy base. If you're lactose intolerant, almond milk and soy milk are good alternatives.

These are just a few of the great benefits you will receive by incorporating Smoothies into your daily Diet and Lifestyle.

2

Setting Realistic Weight Loss Goals

When beginning a weight loss program, the first step you might take is to create monthly weight loss goals. Deciding how much weight you would like to lose each month is important for setting up a realistic diet and exercise program that will offer you longer lasting, permanent weight loss. It's common knowledge that losing weight too fast can lead to swift weight regain since dieting does stress the body. Setting realistic goals now will help you to keep the weight off later.

Don't Pay Attention to Advertisements

Advertisements for diet products usually begin with a client suggesting that she lost a significant amount of weight very quickly and went from a "size 19 to a size 6!" And while it is definitely possible to lose a significant amount of weight, the timeframes suggested by most diet promotions are quite unrealistic.

No matter your current weight, it is usually a bad idea to lose any more than around 1 pound a week. Although the exact number of calories you need to burn in excess may vary slightly, a 1 pound weekly loss means burning about 5000 calories more than you take in. To put that number into perspective, burning 5000 calories is like a 130 pound female doing 15 hours of aerobics!

If your goal is to lose 50 pounds, realistically, you should aim to lose no more than 1.5 pounds a week. This means about 6 pounds per month and an overall timeframe of approximately 8 months. That might seem like a long time, but losing weight at a slow and steady pace is the best way to keep those pounds off.

Consider the Percentages

The number of pounds you can lose each month and overall can also be influenced by your current weight and how many pounds you would like to lose. A 200 pound female who loses 10 pounds in a month has lost 5% of her bodyweight whereas a 150 pound female who loses 10 pounds in a month has lost 6.5% of her overall bodyweight.

So we can see that the lower your starting weight, the more conservative your monthly weight loss goal should be. In addition, your current weight and weight loss goal should be something to consider each month since a static monthly goal will result in increasingly difficult weight loss should your goals remain too ambitious.

Although your monthly goal might not change significantly, it is important to realize that the closer you come to a weight loss goal, the slower your weight loss may be.

Realize That Every Body is Different

Teaming up with a weight loss buddy is a great way to keep motivated, but your goals should be created from considering your own weight loss needs - not the needs of a weight-loss partner. If your friend wants to lose 25 pounds and your goal is to lose 50 pounds, be aware that your friend may reach her goal first and that increasing the amount of weight you want to lose each month to match your friend's goal is not a healthy idea.

3

Smoothie Recipes for Cleansing and Detox

Buying organic fruits and vegetables will increase the health benefits of the produce you consume, while minimizing toxins like pesticides. Try finding a local farm or CSA, or join a co-op to reduce the costs of buying organic produce.

Most veggies can be cleaned, cut and prepared a couple days in advance.

Make sure you pre-cut celery, carrots and other items that won't absorb plenty of water in a container with cold water to elongate their shelf life. Wait to cut more fragile/quick-to-brown for example tings like apples and cucumbers until right before you juice. Wash everything thoroughly, too!

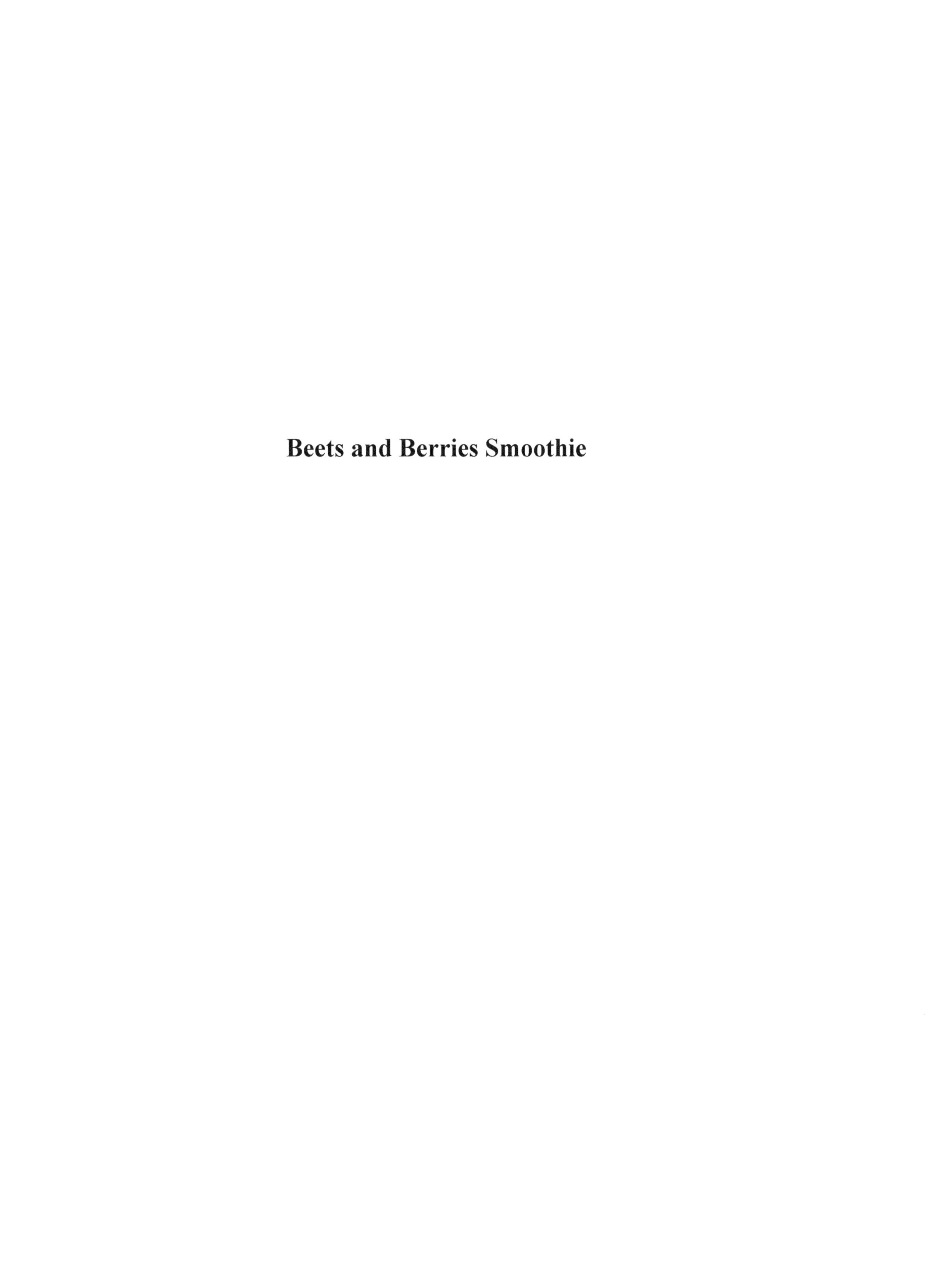

Beets and Berries Smoothie

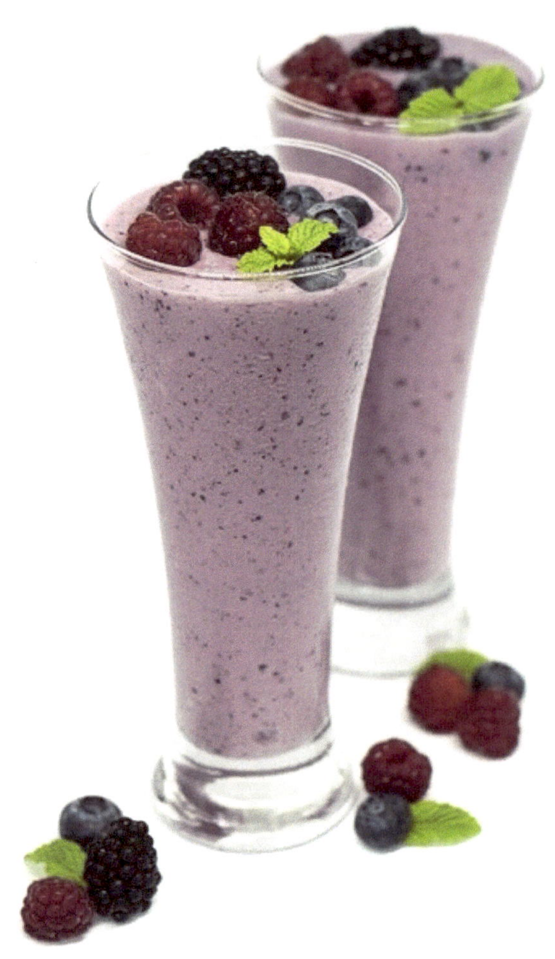

A nourishing smoothie with the sweetness of berries and the cleansing qualities of beetroot. This smoothie will fill you up during your detox and make you glow from the inside out. Filled with antioxidants, iron, good fats and a little zest from the lemon!

Ingredients:
 1 beet

10 strawberries Juice of 1/2 a lemon

1/2 cup coconut milk

3/4 cup coconut water

Directions: Add ingredients to the blender and blend it until its smooth

Super Mint Banana Smoothie

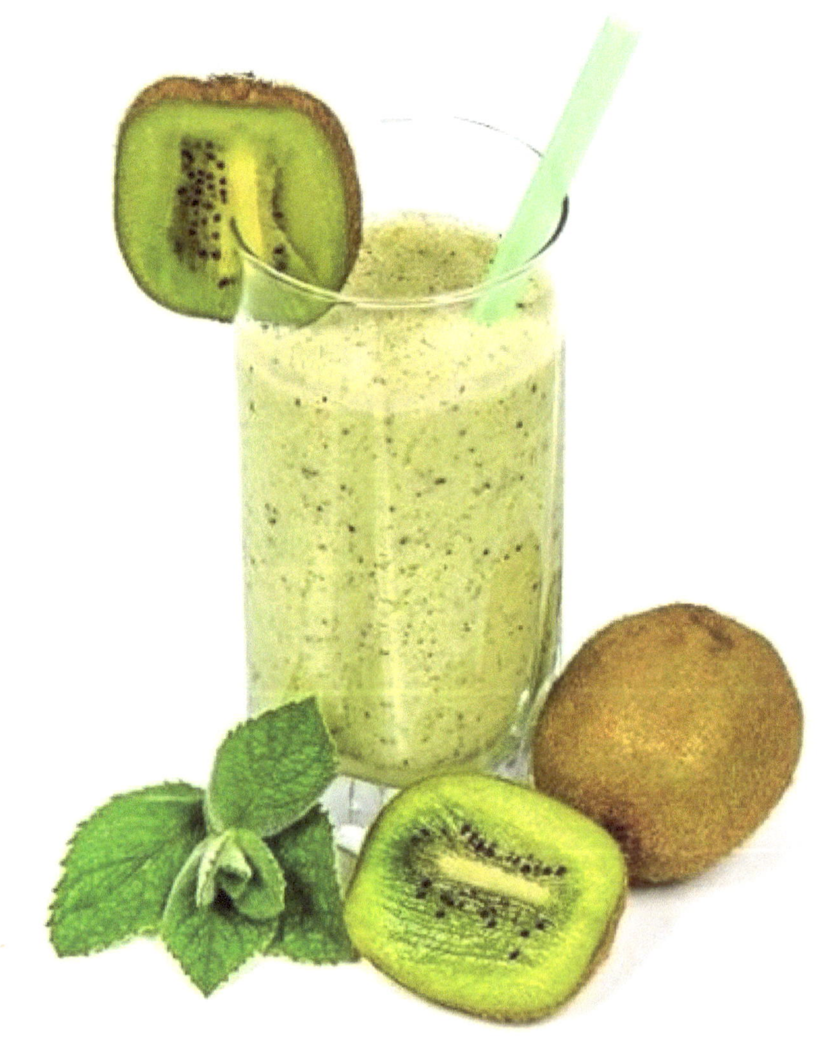

This smoothie has the works! High in fiber and protein to keep your energy levels up for longer. It's also got great sources of good quality fats like omega-3's and mono-unsaturated fats from avocado.

Ingredients:

1 ½ banana

2 teaspoon spirulina

¼ avocado

1 ½ cup almond milk

2 teaspoon chia seeds

2 leaves of kale

1 date

½ cup tightly packed spinach

4-6 drops peppermint extract

Directions: Add ingredients to blender and blend until smooth

Matcha Green Smoothie

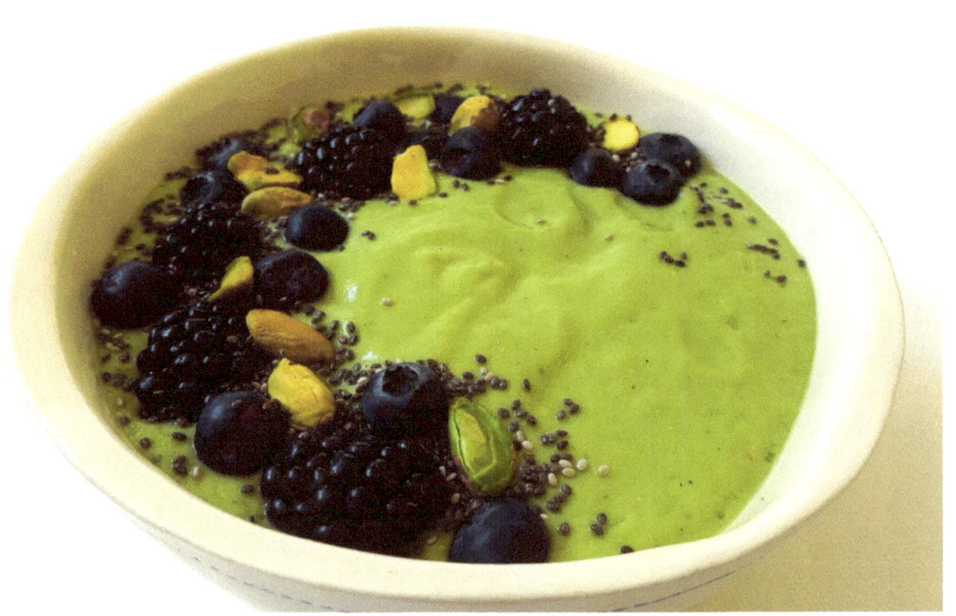

Get your greens with the amazing antioxidant benefits of green tea powder. Matcha is also a great alternative to coffee as it will still give you a boost but is not as strong and intense as coffee.

Ingredients:

3/4 cup almond milk ¾ cup ice

2 tsp honey

1/3 cup soaked cashews

2 tsp matcha powder

½ cup tightly packed spinach

2 tsp coconut cream ½ tsp nutmeg

Directions: Blend all ingredients until smooth

Blood Detox Smoothie

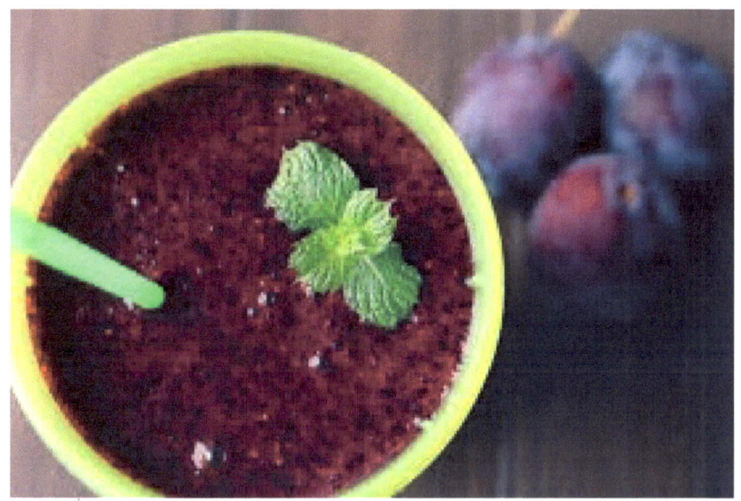

Beet is normally used in many detox smoothie recipes because its one of natures finest!

They are a fantastic source of iron, potassium and antioxidants.

Beets are also great for detoxification thanks to the phytonutrients they contain. The addition of the superfood turmeric to this juice also makes it an anti-inflammatory powerhouse! Drink up!

Ingredients:

4 medium beets

1 orange 2 inches fresh turmeric root What to do

Directions: Juice all ingredients and enjoy

4

Smoothie Recipes for More Energy

Vitamin C Packed Smoothie

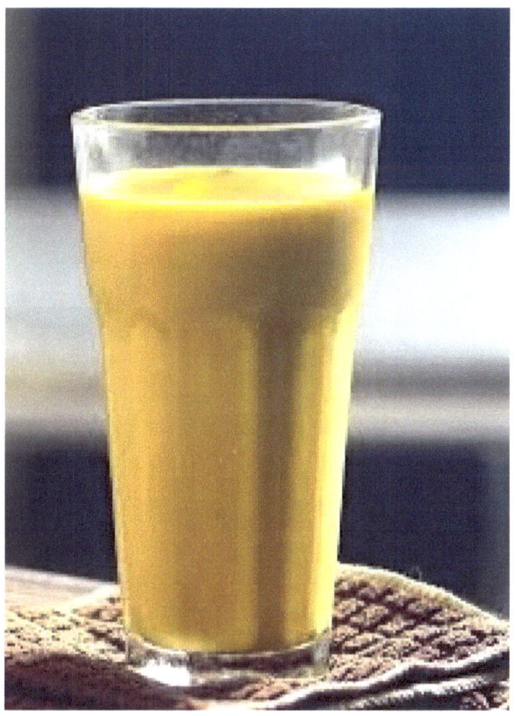

Packed with vitamin C, this sweet and tangy citrus smoothie will inspire smiles on even the rainiest morning.

Ingredients:

2-3 freshly-juiced tangerines

1 ruby red grapefruit (juiced)

A handful of frozen strawberries

Directions:

Peel and juice the tangerines with the grapefruit, and puree the blended juice with the frozen strawberries.

Mango Blueberry Supreme Smoothie

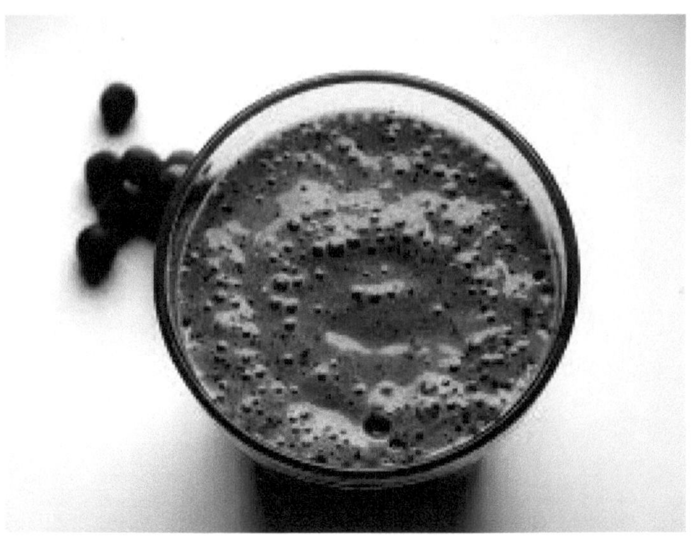

Ingredients:

1 mango, peeled and cubed

1 pint of blueberries

1 banana (frozen or fresh)

1 teaspoon of maple syrup.

1 cup non-dairy milk of choice (almond, soy, or coconut are recommended)

Directions:

Puree all ingredients together in a blender, and enjoy. A handful of chopped ice can be added if desired.

Minty Fruit Cocktail Smoothie

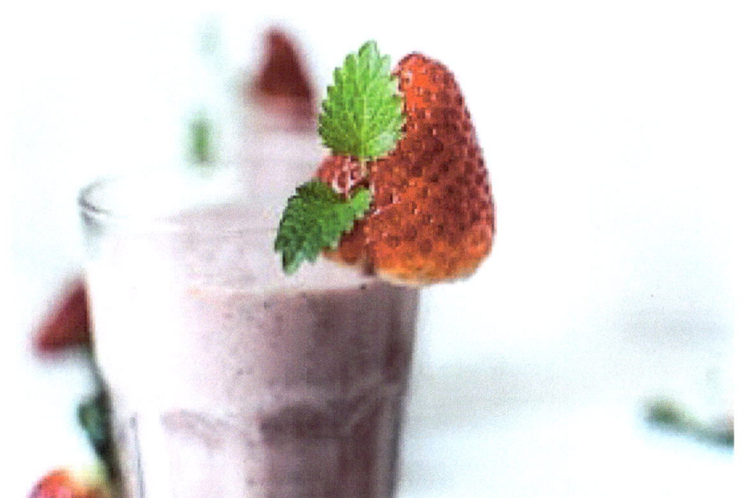

Ingredients:
1 apple, peeled, cored, and sliced

1 orange, peeled and divided

1/2 cup pineapple

2 cups watermelon, cubed and seeded

1 teaspoon lemon juice

A small sprig of fresh mint

Directions:

Juice the apple and orange first, followed by the pineapple. Transfer juice to a blender, and add the watermelon, lemon juice, and mint. Puree until smooth.

Smoothie Recipes For Skin and Hair Care

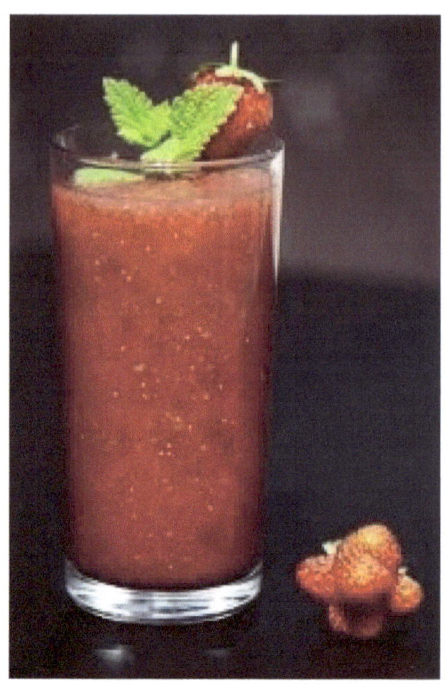

Ingredients:

3 - 5 medium size heirloom tomatoes

1 cup watermelon chunks

1 peach, plum or pear

A handful of mixed herbs like cilantro, basil, watercress, or mint
A touch of red spicy pepper

A touch of sea salt

A handful of sprouted watermelon seeds or pumpkin seeds for crunch
and texture

1 Scoop of Melon

Directions: Blend to desired texture

Tropic Thunder Smoothie

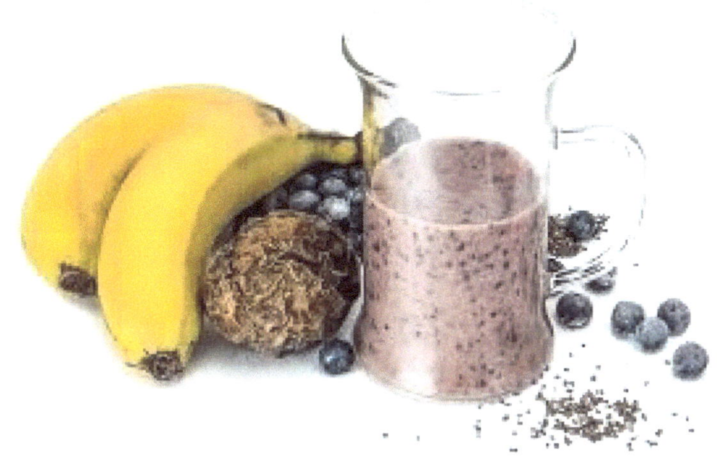

Ingredients:

1 Whole Young Coconut Meat and Coconut Water

1-2 Whole Beets

1 Banana fresh or frozen

Directions:
Place everything into a blender (including whole beets too) and blend for 30 seconds to 1 minute on full speed until blended completely.

Turmeric Cleanser Smoothie

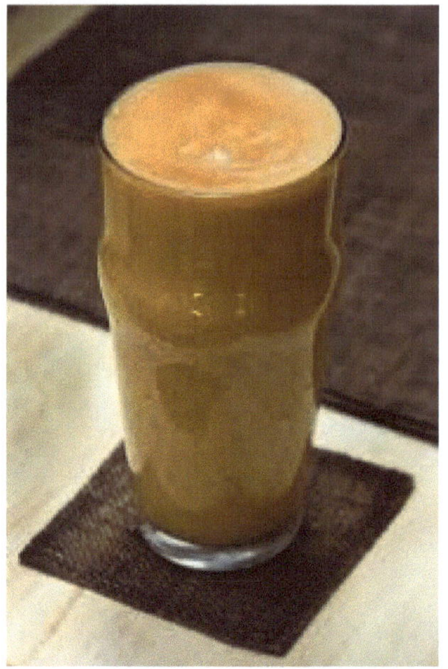

This delicious fruity blend reverses the look of sun damage on your face. Wrinkles, fine lines, dark spots and sagging skin can be transformed, tightened and refreshed by drinking this cleanser just once a day. Turmeric is naturally anti-bacterial and can help ward off cold and flu germs. Also, the high vitamin C content in pineapple gives you another heavy dose of crucial immunity.

Ingredients:
2 full kale, include the stems (I don't Know Why People through this vital part away!?)
¼ cup cilantro
2 cup unsweetened coconut water
2 cup chopped pineapple
1 cup chopped mango
Juice of ½ lemon
½ teaspoon ground turmeric
Directions:
1. Blend kale, cilantro, and coconut water until smooth.
2. Add pineapple, mango, lemon juice, and turmeric and blend a second time.

Kiwi Mint Goddess Smoothie

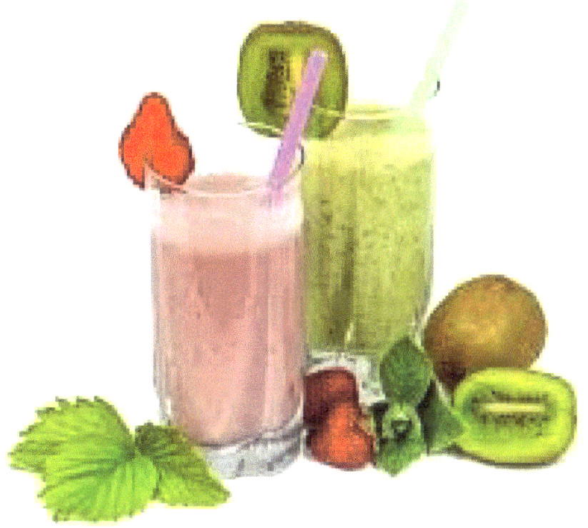

Detox the delicious way with this unique and savory mixture! This smoothie flushes away toxins embedded in the skin to reveal clearer, cleaner and more vibrant cells. The antioxidant content helps strengthen nails, bones and teeth. Don't forget that this particular blend of fruits is amazing for curing digestive upsets and keeping your system running smoothly.

Ingredients:

1½ c spinach

½ c fresh mint leaves

2 c unsweetened coconut water

2 c blackberries

2 kiwifruit, halved

Directions

1. Blend spinach, mint, and coconut water until smooth.

2. Add blackberries and kiwifruit and blend again.

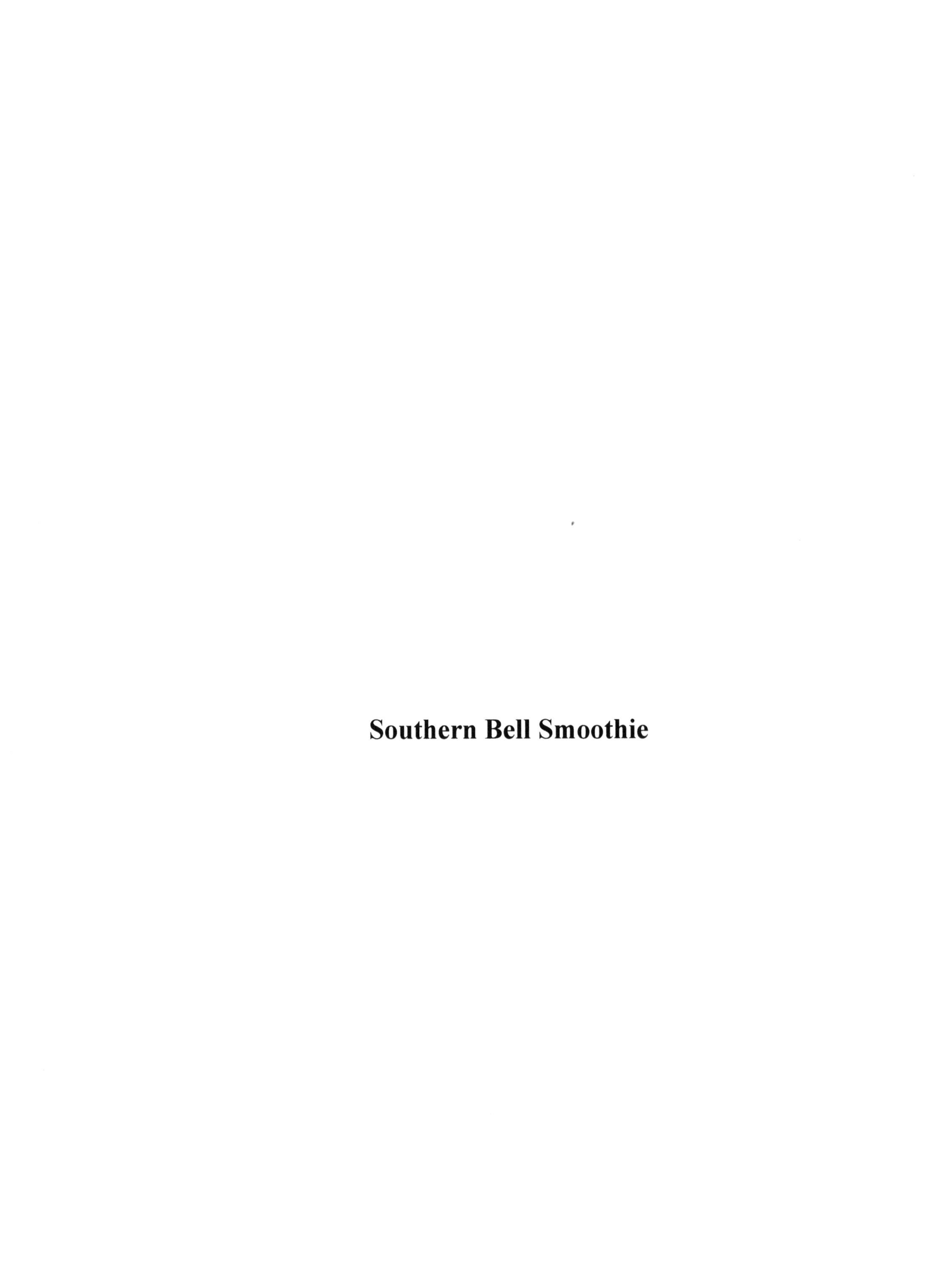

Southern Bell Smoothie

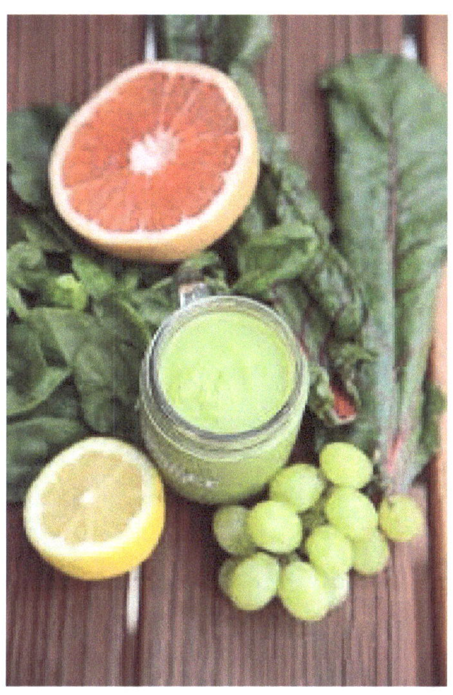

This smoothie is Fantastic! Collard greens, lush cantaloupe and carrots all work together to clean up skin imperfections like blemishes and clogged pores. They also help grow long, strong nails and HEAL, damaged hair follicles.

Ingredients:

2 cup collard greens

1 cup water

1 cup chopped cantaloupe

2 cup chopped mango

½ cup chopped carrots

½ cup chopped pineapple

Directions

1. Blend collard greens, water, and cantaloupe until smooth.

2. Add mango, carrots, and pineapple and blend again.

Smoothie Recipes For Acne

Super Earth Propolis Smoothie

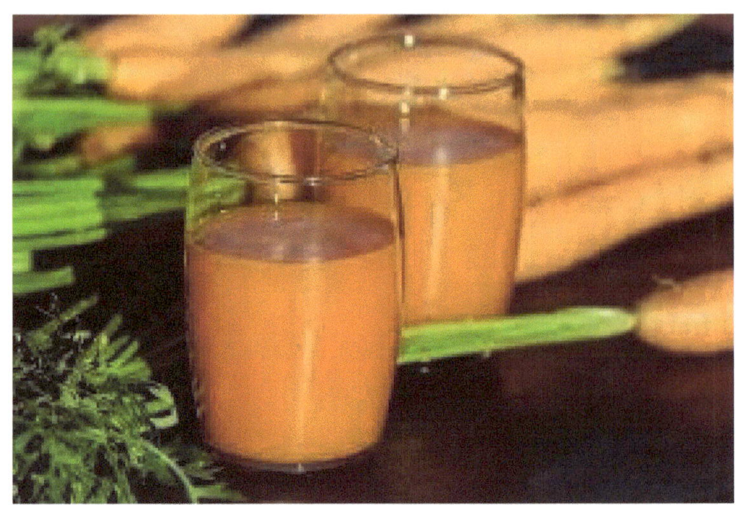

Ingredients:

1 tablespoon Coconut Oil

5 Drops of Propolis – A reddish-brown resinous substance collected by honeybees
 (I like the brand they sell on Amazon by "NOW")

1 whole avocado

7 large carrots- Yes this is Intense, but extremely good for you!

1 small container of blackberries

Directions:
Blend ingredients together and enjoy!

Pumpkin Seed Fennel Smoothie

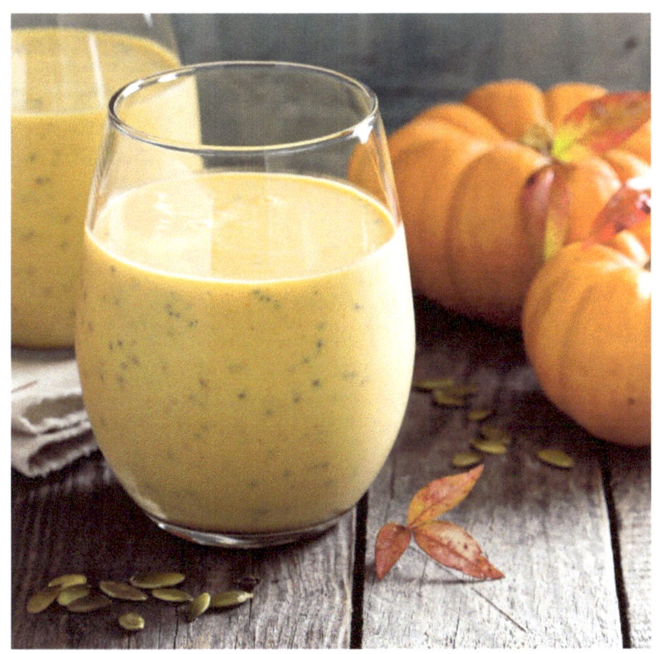

Ingredients:

1 Green Apple

2 tablespoons of raw and unsalted pumpkin seeds

1 sprig of fennel (or a few cuttings)

1 whole avocado

1 thumb of ginger

2 tablespoons of raw and unsalted Almonds – Almonds contain selenium which is good for fighting acne.

Directions: blend all ingredients together and enjoy!

Super Green Avocado Smoothie

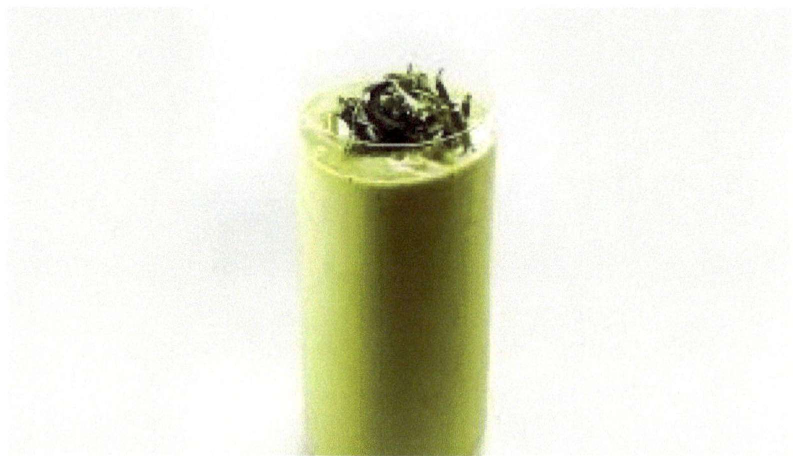

This smoothie packs quite an acne-fighting punch, featuring both avocados and carrots. It even includes blueberries to further boost its antioxidant content, making it one incredibly healthy smoothie overall.

Ingredients:

1 cup spinach

1 carrot

¼ avocado

½ banana

½ pear, cored

½ cup blueberries

1 ½ cups unsweetened almond milk

Directions: Blend All Ingredients together for desired consistency. Enjoy!

Smoothie Recipes for Weight Loss

The key to a successful weight loss journey is starting small - making small realistic changes to your diet or lifestyle until those changes become habits. Rather than attempting to introduce a hundred and one changes at once, get comfortable with one or two new routines before taking on another.
Introducing a well-balanced breakfast smoothie into your day can be an effective way to establish a healthy morning habit, which will in turn have a positive effect on the rest of your day.

We make that transition easy, delivering all the ingredients you need to make healthy smoothies for weight loss at home.

Once you've settled into a healthy breakfast routine, try incorporating some regular exercises, like 25 minutes of walking each day, so you can easily achieve the 150 minutes of recommended exercise per week.

Starting your weight loss journey with a positive mindset and enjoying the experience that comes with trying new combinations of seasonal smoothie ingredients will ultimately support you in sustaining the weight loss. Establishing positive associations with the positive changes you are making in your life will make these changes easier to maintain after you reach your ideal weight.

Making smoothies at home is the easiest way to increase the nutrient density of your meals. When you Opt for less processed foods and eliminate refined sugars and trans fats, it is also wise to make good whole food choices as well. Some of my favorite nutrient-dense ingredients to add to smoothies for weight loss include avocados, leafy greens, bananas, berries, nuts, seeds and super-food powders like cacao and acai.

When it comes to weight loss, burning more calories than you consume is the winning formula. Making smoothies at home gives you the flexibility to alter the calorie count of your smoothies and experiment with different ingredients to understand what your body responds best to.

If you're following a calorie-controlled diet, smoothies are often recommended for breakfast as they serve as a low calorie meal option that can be tailored to your unique needs. For example, to reduce the calories of your smoothie, you can use almond milk, coconut water or even water instead of dairy milk. Or if you would like to increase the protein content of your breakfast, you can add a protein powder to your smoothies every morning.

Tips For Using Smoothies For Weight Loss

- If you want to follow a sustainable smoothie diet plan, start your day with a smoothie for breakfast and have a regular meal for lunch and dinner with a large serving of greens and protein to keep your hunger levels under control.

- Change up your smoothie ingredients so you get a varied source of nutrients

- Try using new combinations of super-foods and smoothies to create well balanced breakfast smoothies and ensure you never get sick of the same old smoothie recipe

- Use fresh, seasonal ingredients wherever possible - avoid canned fruit as this is often preserved in fruit juice

- Avoid sweetened yogurt and milk with artificial colors, flavors, or other additives - natural smoothies for weight loss are the way to go

- Want to make vegan smoothies for weight loss? Use water, coconut water or nut milk instead of dairy based milk.

- Share your favorite smoothie recipes and progress with friends and family to keep you motivated and on track

The Importance of Acai and Blueberry Based Smoothies

Berries are excellent in smoothies for weight loss and for supporting your overall health because they're rich in antioxidants, high in fiber and can support blood sugar levels and regulation.

Packed with powerful antioxidants, protein and essential fatty acids, acai powder is key for crafting energizing breakfast smoothies for weight loss.

And the combination of sunflower and lin-seed takes this healthy smoothie recipe to the next level – super-rich in protein and other essential nutrients, such as copper, vitamin B1, manganese, magnesium, phosphorus and selenium, these super seeds come together to support a healthy heart and immune system

SMOOTHIE RECIPES

Acai Blueberry Smoothie

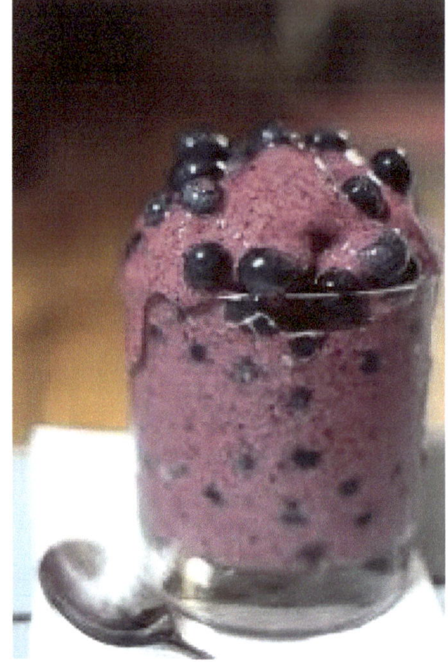

Ingredients:

1 banana

1 handful of blueberries

1 apple (optional)

1 Tbs acai powder

1 Tbs sunflower seeds

1 Tbs linseed

Directions: Blend Ingredients together to desired consistency. Enjoy!

The Lean Belly Smoothie

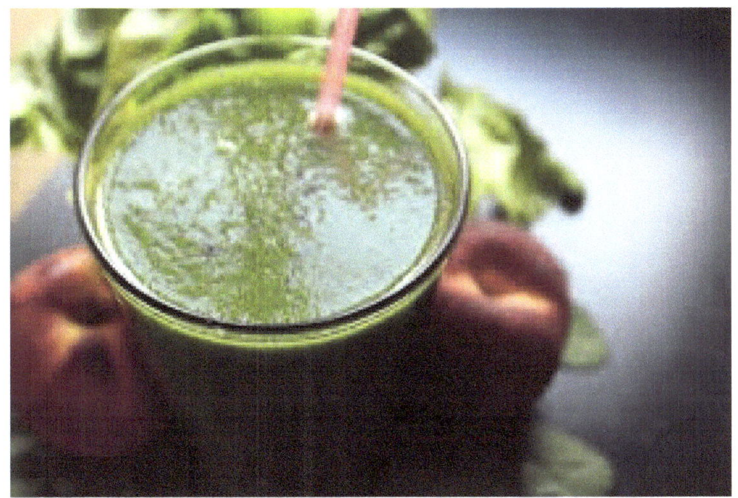

Ingredients:

2 Cups Spinach

½ red grapefruit peeled

½ cup mixed frozen berries

2 table spoon Greek yoghurt

1 table spoon chia seeds

1 cup filtered water

Directions: Blend All Ingredients together and enjoy!

Berry Fit Smoothie

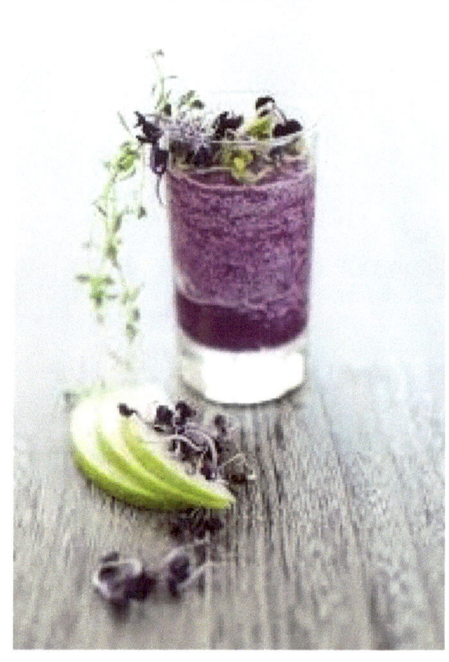

Ingredients:

3 ounces vanilla Greek yogurt

1 tablespoon almond butter

1/2 cup frozen blueberries

1/2 cup frozen pineapple

1 cup kale

3/4 cup water

Directions: Blend All Ingredients together for desired consistency. Enjoy!

Super Kale Blaster Smoothie

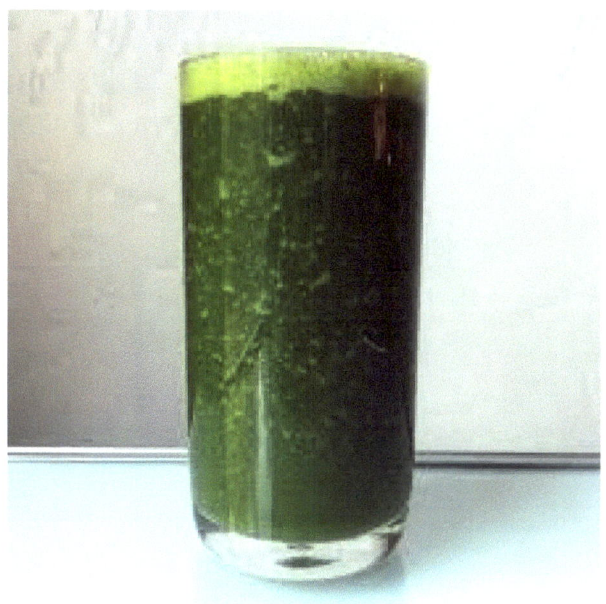

Ingredients:

2 cups kale

1 cup spinach

3 bannas

½ cup blueberries

1 teaspoon of chia seeds

Directions: Blend All Ingredients together and enjoy!

Dinosaur Kale Smoothie

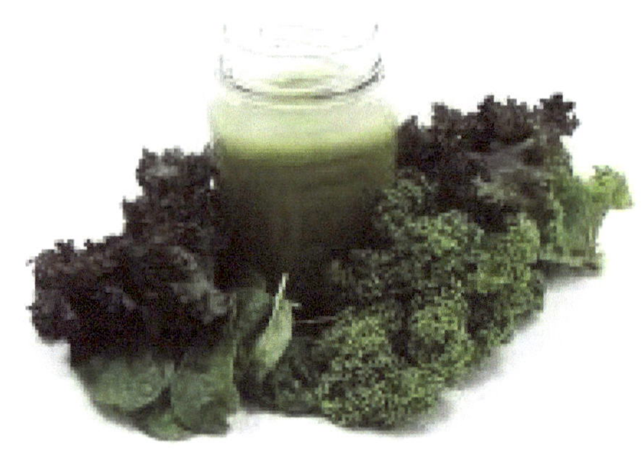

Ingredients:

½ cup of Greek Yogurt
1 whole bushel of dinosaur kale
1 tablespoon of coconut oil
1 whole avocado
2 green apples
½ cup blackberries
½ lemon

Directions: Blend All Ingredients together including the stems from the dinosaur kale. Enjoy!

Almond Butter Buster Smoothie

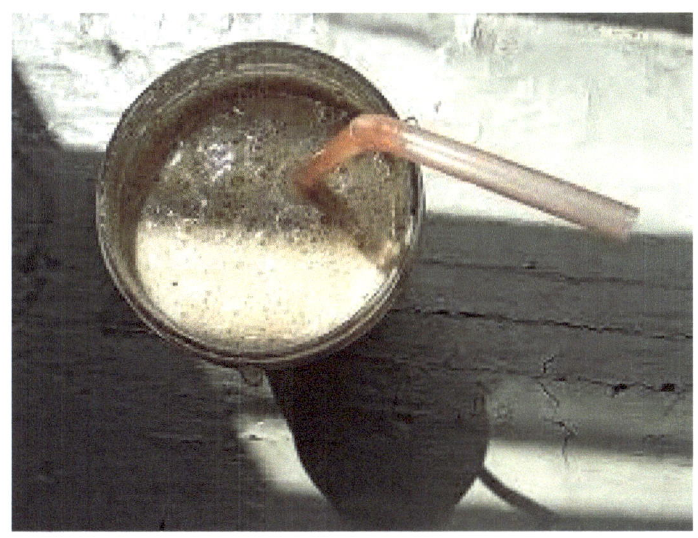

Ingredients:

2 Bananas

1 cup almond milk

3 tablespoons almond butter

1 tablespoon ground flax seed

Directions: Blend All ingredients to desired consistency. Enjoy!

Mango Refresher Smoothie

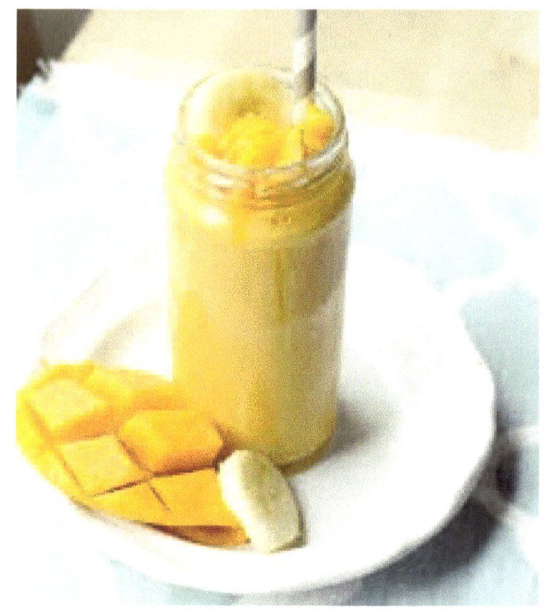

Ingredients:

¼ cup mango cubes

¼ cup mashed ripe avocado

½ cup mango juice

¼ cup fat-free vanilla yogurt

1 Tablespoon freshly squeezed lime-juice

1 Tablespoon sugar

6 ice cubes

Directions: Blend all ingredients in a blender to gain desired consistency.
Enjoy!

Conclusion

We hope you enjoyed reading SkinnyGal Smoothies. It is our hope that the smoothie recipes in this book will help individuals who desire to enhance their diets and lose weight using Natural alternatives, such as whole foods. Smoothies can be very powerful in health, fitness, vitality, and your energy.

Thank You and Good Luck on Your Journey!